The Senior Stretch Handbook

Easy, Effective Exercises for Improved Mobility and Quality of Life

Clara Winter

Copyrights © Clara Winter

This content contain within this book may not be reproduced, duplicated or transmitted without direct permission from the Author or the publisher.

Table of Contents

Introduction

Welcome to "The Senior Stretch Handbook: Easy, Effective Exercises for Improved Mobility and Quality of Life"! In this book, we will be exploring a variety of stretching exercises and techniques that are specifically tailored to the needs and abilities of seniors.

As we age, it's natural for our bodies to lose some of their flexibility and mobility. However, maintaining a regular stretching routine can help to slow down this process and even improve our physical function and overall quality of life. Stretching can also provide numerous other benefits, including improved balance and posture, reduced risk of falls, and relief from common senior ailments such as back pain and arthritis.

So, why is stretching so important for seniors? As we age, our muscles tend to shorten and become tighter, which can lead to a decrease in range of motion and an increased risk of injury. Stretching helps to lengthen and loosen these muscles, improving our ability to move freely and comfortably. It can also help to improve our balance and coordination, which can be especially beneficial for seniors who are at a higher risk of falls.

But stretching aren't just about physical benefits. It can also have a positive impact on our mental and emotional well-being. Stretching can help to reduce stress and improve relaxation, and it can be a great way to incorporate mindfulness and meditation into our daily routines.

So, now that we understand the importance of stretching for seniors, let's get started! In the following chapters, we will be covering a range of stretching exercises that can be easily incorporated into any senior's routine, regardless of fitness level or mobility. We will also be exploring advanced stretching techniques and the role of props and tools, as well as how to safely progress and increase the intensity of your stretches as you gain flexibility and strength.

So grab your stretch band or yoga mat and let's get started on improving your flexibility, mobility, and overall quality of life!

Chapter One

The Importance of Maintaining Flexibility and Mobility as We Age

Maintaining flexibility and mobility is crucial for seniors for a number of reasons. As we age, our muscles naturally shorten and become tighter, which can lead to a decrease in range of motion and an increased risk of injury. This can make it more difficult to perform everyday activities such as reaching, bending, and walking, and it can also contribute to feelings of stiffness and discomfort.

However, maintaining a regular stretching routine can help to slow down the natural process of muscle tightening and improve our range of motion. It can also help to improve our balance and coordination, which can be especially beneficial for seniors who are at a higher risk of falls. In addition, stretching can help to alleviate common senior ailments such as back pain and arthritis, as well as improve posture and reduce the risk of developing poor posture.

Overall, maintaining flexibility and mobility is essential for seniors in order to remain independent, active, and able to perform daily tasks comfortably and safely. By incorporating stretching into your routine, you can enjoy the many physical and mental benefits that come with staying limber and agile as you age.

The benefits of stretching for seniors, including improved balance, posture, and physical function

Benefits of Stretching for Seniors

Improved balance and coordination

Stretching helps to lengthen and loosen tight muscles, which can improve balance and coordination. This is especially important for seniors, who may be at a higher risk of falls due to decreased muscle strength and balance.

Improved posture

Tight muscles can contribute to poor posture, which can lead to a range of issues such as back pain and discomfort. Stretching can help to improve posture by lengthening tight muscles and strengthening supportive muscles.

Improved physical function

Stretching can help to improve range of motion, making it easier to perform everyday tasks such as reaching, bending, and walking. It can also help to alleviate common senior ailments such as back pain and arthritis, which can improve overall physical function.

Stress relief and relaxation

Stretching can be a great way to reduce stress and improve relaxation. It can be especially beneficial for seniors who may be experiencing increased stress or anxiety due to the challenges of aging.

Improved mental and emotional well-being

In addition to its physical benefits, stretching can also have a positive impact on mental and emotional well-being. Incorporating mindful breathing and meditation into a stretching routine can help to improve focus and calm the mind.

Overall, incorporating stretching into your routine can provide a range of physical and mental benefits that can help to improve your quality of life as you age.

How to get started with a stretching routine

Starting a stretching routine is easy and can be done by anyone, regardless of age or fitness level. Here are some tips to help you get started:

Consult with your healthcare provider

It's always a good idea to consult with your healthcare provider before starting a new exercise routine, especially if you have any pre-existing health conditions. They can help you to determine the types of stretches that are safe and appropriate for you, and they can also provide guidance on how often and how intensely you should be stretching.

Find a comfortable, quiet space

Choose a quiet, comfortable space where you can stretch without distractions. This could be a quiet corner of your living room, a yoga studio, or even your backyard. Just be sure to choose a space where you feel comfortable and relaxed.

Gather your supplies

Depending on the type of stretches you'll be doing, you may need a few supplies such as a yoga mat, stretch band, or foam roller. Gather these supplies before you get started so that you have everything you need on hand.

Warm up before stretching

It's important to warm up your muscles before stretching to help prevent injury. Try taking a brief walk or doing some light calisthenics such as arm circles or leg swings to get your blood flowing.

Start with basic stretches

Begin with basic stretches that are easy and comfortable for you. As you gain flexibility and strength, you can gradually progress to more advanced stretches.

Hold stretches for at least 30 seconds

To get the most benefit from your stretches, hold each stretch for at least 30 seconds. If you're able to, try holding the stretch for up to a minute.

Stretch both sides

Be sure to stretch both sides of your body evenly to maintain balance.

Stretch regularly

To get the most benefit from stretching, aim to stretch at least a few times a week. You can also try incorporating stretching into your daily routine by doing a few stretches when you wake up in the morning and before you go to bed at night.

Remember to listen to your body and stop if you feel any pain or discomfort. Stretching should be a comfortable and enjoyable activity, not a source of pain or discomfort. With regular practice, you'll soon be reaping the many benefits that stretching has to offer.

Chapter 2

Upper Body Stretches

We will be exploring a variety of upper body stretches that can help to improve flexibility and mobility in the neck, shoulders, arms, and wrists. These stretches are gentle and easy to do, and they can be modified to suit your individual flexibility and comfort level.

Neck stretches

Tightness in the neck can lead to discomfort and difficulty turning your head. To stretch the neck, try the following:

Neck tilt stretch

Slowly tilt your head to one side, bringing your ear towards your shoulder. Hold for 30 seconds, then switch sides.

Neck rotation stretch

Slowly turn your head to one side, bringing your chin towards your shoulder. Hold for 30 seconds, then switch sides.

Neck side bend stretch

Slowly bend your head to one side, bringing your ear towards your shoulder. Hold for 30 seconds, then switch sides.

Shoulder stretches

Tight shoulders can lead to discomfort and difficulty reaching overhead. To stretch the shoulders, try the following:

Shoulder roll stretch

Roll your shoulders backwards and forwards, slowly and gently.

Shoulder blade squeeze stretch

Squeeze your shoulder blades together and hold for 30 seconds, then release.

Arm across chest stretch

Hold one arm across your chest with the opposite hand, and gently pull the arm in towards your chest until you feel a stretch in the shoulder. Hold for 30 seconds, then switch sides.

Arm and wrist stretch

Tightness in the arms and wrists can make it difficult to perform tasks such as typing and writing. To stretch the arms and wrists, try the following:

Arm and wrist stretch

Hold one arm out in front of you with your palm facing down. Gently bend your wrist down and hold for 30 seconds, then switch sides.

Triceps stretch

Hold one arm behind your back with your palm facing up. Gently use your opposite hand to gently push your elbow down towards your back until you feel a stretch in the triceps. Hold for 30 seconds, then switch sides.

Remember to breathe deeply and relax as you hold each stretch. As you gain flexibility, you can hold each stretch for longer periods of time and try to increase the intensity of the stretch. Just be sure to listen to your body and stop if you feel any pain or discomfort.

Chest stretch

Stand with your arms behind your back, palms facing each other. Gently lift your arms up and back until you feel a stretch in your chest. Hold for 30 seconds.

Overhead reach stretch

Stand with your arms by your sides and your feet shoulder-width apart. Reach one arm up overhead, keeping the other arm by your side. Hold for 30 seconds, then switch sides.

Cross body arm stretch

Stand with your arms by your sides and your feet shoulder-width apart. Reach one arm across your body, holding onto the opposite elbow with the other hand. Hold for 30 seconds, then switch sides.

Wrist flexor stretch

Hold one arm out in front of you with your palm facing down. Use your other hand to gently press down on the back of your hand until you feel a stretch in your wrist. Hold for 30 seconds, then switch sides.

Wrist extensor stretch

Hold one arm out in front of you with your palm facing up. Use your other hand to gently press down on the top of your hand until you feel a stretch in your wrist. Hold for 30 seconds, then switch sides.

Remember to be gentle and avoid overstretching. If you feel any pain or discomfort, stop the stretch and try a modified version. With regular practice, these upper body stretches can help to improve flexibility and mobility in the neck, shoulders, arms, and wrists.

Chapter 3

Lower Body Stretches

We will be exploring a variety of lower body stretches that can help to improve flexibility and mobility in the legs, hips, and ankles. These stretches are gentle and easy to do, and they can be modified to suit your individual flexibility and comfort level.

Leg stretches

Tightness in the legs can lead to discomfort and difficulty walking or climbing stairs. To stretch the legs, try the following:

Hamstring stretch

Stand with your feet shoulder-width apart and extend one leg out in front of you. Bend forward at the waist and try to touch your toes, keeping your back straight. Hold for 30 seconds, then switch sides.

Quadricep stretch

Stand with your feet shoulder-width apart and bend one leg behind you, holding onto your ankle with your hand. Gently pull your heel towards your butt until you feel a stretch in the front of your thigh. Hold for 30 seconds, then switch sides.

Calf stretch

Stand facing a wall and place one foot behind you, keeping the heel on the ground and the toes pointed towards the wall. Lean into the wall until you feel a stretch in your calf. Hold for 30 seconds, then switch sides.

Hip stretches

Tightness in the hips can lead to discomfort and difficulty standing for long periods of time. To stretch the hips, try the following:

Hip flexor stretch

Stand with your feet shoulder-width apart and bring one foot up behind you, placing your foot on a bench or chair. Lean forward slightly until you feel a stretch in the front of your hip. Hold for 30 seconds, then switch sides.

Glute stretches

Sit on the ground with both legs extended in front of you. Cross one ankle over the opposite knee and gently press down on the bent knee until you feel a stretch in the glute. Hold for 30 seconds, then switch sides.

Ankle and foot stretches

Tightness in the ankles and feet can lead to discomfort and difficulty walking or standing for long periods of time. To stretch the ankles and feet, try the following:

Ankle rotation stretch

Sit on the ground with both legs extended in front of you. Lift one leg off the ground and gently rotate the ankle in a circular motion. Do 10-15 rotations in each direction, then switch sides.

Foot stretch

Sit on the ground with both legs extended in front of you. Place a towel or band around the ball of one foot and gently pull the foot towards you until you feel a stretch in the foot and ankle. Hold for 30 seconds, then switch sides.

Remember to breathe deeply and relax as you hold each stretch. As you gain flexibility, you can hold each stretch for longer periods of time and try to increase the intensity of the stretch. Just be sure to listen to your body and stop if you feel any pain or discomfort.

Chapter 4

Stretching for Common Senior Ailments

As we age, it's natural for our bodies to experience some aches and pains. However, regular stretching can help to alleviate many common senior ailments and improve overall physical function. In this chapter, we will be exploring stretches that can be particularly helpful for relieving back pain, improving mobility in the knees and hips, and relieving chronic conditions such as arthritis and fibromyalgia.

Stretches for back pain

Back pain is a common issue for seniors, and it can be caused by a variety of factors such as poor posture, muscle imbalances, and degenerative conditions. To help alleviate back pain, try the following stretches:

Cat-cow stretch

Start on all fours with your hands under your shoulders and your knees under your hips. Inhale as you round your spine and tuck your chin towards your chest (cat position). Exhale as you arch your back and look up towards the ceiling (cow position). Repeat for 5-10 reps.

Child's pose stretch

Start on all fours with your hands under your shoulders and your knees under your hips. Slowly lower your hips back towards your heels and stretch your arms out in front of you. Hold for 30 seconds.

Spinal twist stretch

Sit on the ground with both legs extended in front of you. Cross one leg over the other and gently twist your upper body towards the bent leg. Hold for 30 seconds, then switch sides.

Stretches for the knees and hips

As we age, it's common for the knees and hips to become stiff and painful. To help improve mobility and reduce pain in these areas, try the following stretches:

Knee to chest stretch

Lie on your back with both legs extended. Bring one knee towards your chest and hold it with both hands. Gently press down on the bent knee to increase the stretch, and hold for 30 seconds. Switch sides and repeat.

Pigeon pose stretch

Start on all fours with your hands under your shoulders and your knees under your hips. Bring one leg forward and bend the knee, placing the ankle just outside of the opposite hip. Slowly lower your hips towards the ground until you feel a stretch in the hip and thigh. Hold for 30 seconds, then switch sides.

Lunge stretch

Step one foot forward and bend the front knee, keeping the back knee straight and the heel on the ground. Gently lean forward until you feel a stretch in the front of the back leg. Hold for 30 seconds, then switch sides.

Stretches for chronic conditions

Chronic conditions such as arthritis and fibromyalgia can cause widespread pain and stiffness. To help alleviate symptoms, try the following stretches:

Neck tilt stretch

Slowly tilt your head to one side, bringing your ear towards your shoulder. Hold for 30 seconds, then switch sides.

Shoulder blade squeeze stretch

Squeeze your shoulder blades together and hold for 30 seconds, then release.

Chest stretch

Stand with your arms behind your back, palms facing each other. Gently lift your arms up and back until you feel a stretch in your chest. Hold for 30 seconds.

Hamstring stretch

Stand with your feet shoulder-width apart and extend one leg out in front of you. Bend forward at the waist and try to touch your toes, keeping your back straight. Hold for 30 seconds, then switch sides.

Calf stretch

Stand facing a wall and place one foot behind you, keeping the heel on the ground and the toes pointed towards the wall. Lean into the wall until you feel a stretch in your calf. Hold for 30 seconds, then switch sides.

Glute stretches

Sit on the ground with both legs extended in front of you. Cross one ankle over the opposite knee and gently press down on the bent knee until you feel a stretch in the glute. Hold for 30 seconds, then switch sides.

Remember to listen to your body and only do stretches that feel comfortable for you. It's important to avoid overstretching or forcing your body into positions that cause pain. With regular practice, these stretches can help to alleviate common senior ailments and improve overall physical function.

Chapter 5

Stretching for Improved Balance and Coordination

As we age, it's natural for our balance and coordination to decline. However, regular stretching can help to improve these important skills, reducing the risk of falls and improving overall physical function. In this chapter, we will be exploring stretches that can help to improve balance and coordination, particularly for seniors.

Leg and core strengthening stretches

Strong legs and a stable core are essential for good balance. To improve these areas, try the following stretches:

Squats

Stand with your feet shoulder-width apart and lower yourself down into a squat position, keeping your weight in your heels. Stand back up and repeat for 10-15 reps.

Lunges

Step one foot forward and bend the front knee, keeping the back knee straight and the heel on the ground. Gently lean forward until you feel a stretch in the front of the back leg. Stand back up and repeat for 10-15 reps on each side.

Planks

Start on all fours with your hands under your shoulders and your knees under your hips. Lower yourself down onto your forearms and extend your legs out behind you, keeping your body in a straight line. Hold for 30 seconds, then release.

Balance-specific stretches

Improving balance involves more than just leg and core strength. It also requires good proprioception (awareness of the position of your body in space) and coordination. To improve these skills, try the following stretches:

Single leg balance

Stand on one leg with your arms at your sides. Hold for 30 seconds, then switch sides.

Heel-to-toe walk

Walk forward, placing one foot directly in front of the other so that the heel of the front foot touches the toes of the back foot. Walk for 10 steps, then turn around and walk back.

Tandem walk

Walk forward, placing one foot directly in front of the other so that the heel of the front foot touches the toes of the back foot. Focus on a point in front of you to help improve your balance. Walk for 10 steps, then turn around and walk back.

Stretches to improve coordination

Good coordination involves the ability to smoothly and accurately move your body through space. To improve coordination, try the following stretches:

Arm circles

Stand with your arms by your sides and slowly make circular movements with your arms, first in one direction and then in the other.

Leg swings

Stand facing a wall and gently swing one leg forwards and backwards, keeping your foot relaxed. Do 10-15 swings in each direction, then switch sides.

Marching in place

Stand with your arms by your sides and lift one knee up towards your chest, then gently lower it back down. Alternate legs and march in place for 30 seconds.

Remember to start slowly and gradually increase the difficulty of these stretches as you improve. It's important to listen to your body and only do stretches that feel comfortable for you. With regular practice, these stretches can help to improve balance and coordination, reducing the risk of falls and improving overall physical function.

Chapter 6

Stretching on the Go: Tips for Incorporating Stretches into Your Daily Routine

Stretching is an important part of maintaining flexibility and mobility, and it's something that can be easily incorporated into your daily routine. Here are a few tips for stretching on the go:

Take breaks throughout the day

If you spend a lot of time sitting or standing in one position, it's important to take breaks and stretch your muscles. Even just a few minutes of stretching can help to alleviate tension and improve circulation.

Find stretches that can be done anytime, anywhere: There are many stretches that can be done without any special equipment or a dedicated space. Try stretches such as neck tilts, shoulder rolls, and leg swings that can be done standing or sitting.

Incorporate stretches into your daily routine

There are many opportunities to stretch throughout the day. For example, you can stretch while you're waiting in line, watching TV, or talking on the phone.

Take advantage of natural breaks

If you're out and about, take advantage of natural breaks in your day to stretch. For example, you can stretch while you're waiting for the bus or train, or during a break at work.

Be consistent

The most important thing is to be consistent with your stretching. It's better to do a few stretches every day than to try to do a lot of stretching all at once.

By incorporating stretches into your daily routine, you can maintain flexibility and mobility, and enjoy the many benefits of stretching. So, it's important to make time for stretching, no matter how busy you are.

Stretching exercises that can be done in a chair or seated position

Here are a few stretching exercises that can be done in a chair or seated position:

Neck tilt stretch

Slowly tilt your head to one side, bringing your ear towards your shoulder. Hold for 30 seconds, then switch sides.

Shoulder blade squeeze stretch

Squeeze your shoulder blades together and hold for 30 seconds, then release.

Chest stretch

Sit in a chair and extend your arms out to the sides at shoulder level. Gently press your hands together until you feel a stretch in your chest. Hold for 30 seconds.

Arm circles

Sit in a chair and extend your arms out to the sides at shoulder level. Slowly make circular movements with your arms, first in one direction and then in the other.

Leg swings

Sit in a chair and gently swing one leg forwards and backwards, keeping your foot relaxed. Do 10-15 swings in each direction, then switch sides.

Ankle rotation stretch

Sit in a chair and lift one leg off the ground. Gently rotate the ankle in a circular motion. Do 10-15 rotations in each direction, then switch sides.

Remember to take it easy and only do stretches that feel comfortable for you. With regular practice, these stretches can help to improve flexibility and mobility, even if you are seated.

Chapter 7

Advanced Stretching Techniques: Tips for Improving Flexibility and Mobility

If you're looking to take your stretching to the next level, there are a few advanced techniques you can try. These techniques can help to improve flexibility and mobility, but it's important to approach them with caution and only do stretches that feel comfortable for you.

Proprioceptive neuromuscular facilitation (PNF) stretching

PNF stretching involves actively contracting and relaxing the muscles being stretched. This type of stretching can be very effective, but it should only be done with the guidance of a trained professional.

Static stretching

Static stretching involves holding a stretch for a prolonged period of time, usually 30 seconds or more. This type of stretching can be very effective for increasing flexibility, but it's important to avoid overstretching or forcing your body into positions that cause pain.

Dynamic stretching

Dynamic stretching involves actively moving through a range of motion and is often used as a warm-up before exercise. Examples of dynamic stretches include leg swings and arm circles.

Isometric stretching

Isometric stretching involves contracting the muscles being stretched while also trying to stretch them. This type of stretching can be very effective, but it should be approached with caution and only done with the guidance of a trained professional.

Remember to listen to your body and only do stretches that feel comfortable for you. With regular practice, these advanced stretching techniques can help to improve flexibility and mobility. Just be sure to approach them with caution.

Tips for Increasing the Intensity and Effectiveness of Your Stretches

If you're looking to increase the intensity and effectiveness of your stretches, there are a few things you can try:

Hold stretches for longer periods of time

Static stretches are most effective when they are held for 30 seconds or more. By increasing the duration of your stretches, you can increase the intensity and effectiveness.

Use props

Props such as stretch bands, foam rollers, and yoga blocks can help to increase the intensity of your stretches. These props can provide additional resistance or support, allowing you to stretch deeper into a position.

Gradually increase the intensity

It's important to gradually increase the intensity of your stretches to avoid overstretching or causing injury. Start with a comfortable stretch and gradually increase the intensity over time as you become more flexible.

Warm up before stretching

Warming up before stretching can help to increase the effectiveness of your stretches. Try light cardio or dynamic stretches to get your muscles warmed up before moving into static stretches.

Stretch after exercise

Stretching after exercise can help to increase the effectiveness of your stretches. Your muscles will be warm and more receptive to stretching after a workout.

By following these tips, you can increase the intensity and effectiveness of your stretches and improve flexibility and mobility over time. Remember to listen to your body and only do stretches that feel comfortable for you.

The Role of Props and Tools, such as Yoga Blocks and Straps, in Stretching

Props and tools, such as yoga blocks and straps, can be very helpful in stretching, particularly for those who are new to stretching or have limited flexibility. Here are a few ways that props and tools can be used in stretching:

Yoga blocks

Yoga blocks can be used to support the body and provide additional stability in stretches. For example, you can use a block to support your hands in a forward bend, allowing you to stretch deeper into the position.

Yoga straps

Yoga straps can be used to provide additional resistance in stretches, particularly for stretches that involve the legs. For example, you can use a strap to help you reach your toes in a seated forward bend.

Foam rollers

Foam rollers can be used to provide support and stability in stretches, particularly for stretches that involve the back. For example, you can use a foam roller to support your spine in a stretch such as the cat-cow stretch.

Resistance bands

Resistance bands can provide additional resistance in stretches, allowing you to increase the intensity of your stretches over time. For example, you can use a resistance band to add resistance to stretches such as leg raises or chest presses.

By using props and tools, you can increase the effectiveness of your stretches and make them more accessible, particularly if you are new to stretching or have limited flexibility. Remember to use these props and tools with caution and only do stretches that feel comfortable for you.

How to Safely Progress to More Advanced Stretches as You Gain Flexibility and Strength

As you gain flexibility and strength, you may want to progress to more advanced stretches. Here are a few tips for safely progressing to more advanced stretches:

Gradually increase the intensity of your stretches

It's important to gradually increase the intensity of your stretches to avoid overstretching or causing injury. Start with a comfortable stretch and gradually increase the intensity over time as you become more flexible.

Use props

Props such as yoga blocks and straps can help to support your body and make stretches more accessible, particularly if you are new to stretching or have limited flexibility.

Warm up before stretching

Warming up before stretching can help to increase the effectiveness of your stretches. Try light cardio or dynamic stretches to get your muscles warmed up before moving into static stretches.

Listen to your body

It's important to listen to your body and only do stretches that feel comfortable for you. If a stretch feels painful or uncomfortable, stop immediately and consider trying a different stretch.

Work with a trained professional

If you are unsure about how to safely progress to more advanced stretches, consider working with a trained professional such as a physical therapist or yoga instructor. They can help to guide you and ensure that you are stretching safely and effectively.

By following these tips, you can safely progress to more advanced stretches and continue to improve flexibility and strength over time. Remember to listen to your body and only do stretches that feel comfortable for you.

Chapter 8

Stretching for Mental and Emotional Health: The Surprising Benefits of Stretching

While stretching is often associated with physical benefits such as increased flexibility and mobility, it can also have a positive impact on mental and emotional health.

Ways that Stretching can Benefit your Overall Well-being:

Reduces stress: Stretching can help to reduce stress by releasing tension in the muscles and calming the mind. It's a great way to take a break from the demands of daily life and focus on the present moment.

Improves mood

Stretching can help to improve mood by releasing endorphins, the body's "feel-good" chemicals. It's a simple, yet effective way to boost your mood and improve overall well-being.

Increases mindfulness

Stretching requires you to focus on your breath and the sensation of stretching, which can help to increase mindfulness and improve overall well-being.

Promotes relaxation

Stretching can help to relax the mind and body, making it a great way to unwind after a long day.

By incorporating stretching into your daily routine, you can enjoy the many physical and mental benefits it has to offer. Remember to listen to your body and only do stretches that feel comfortable for you. With regular practice, stretching can help to improve overall well-being and promote a sense of calm and relaxation.

The Link Between Physical and Mental Well-Being: How Taking Care of Your Body Can Benefit Your Mind

It's well-known that physical activity and exercise are important for maintaining physical health, but did you know that they can also have a positive impact on mental well-being? Here are a few ways that taking care of your physical health can benefit your mental health:

Reduces stress

Physical activity and exercise can help to reduce stress by releasing endorphins, the body's "feel-good" chemicals. It's a great way to take a break from the demands of daily life and relax the mind.

Improves mood

Physical activity and exercise can help to improve mood by reducing feelings of anxiety and depression. It's a simple, yet effective way to boost your mood and improve overall well-being.

Increases self-esteem

Engaging in physical activity and exercise can help to increase self-esteem and body confidence. It's a great way to feel good about yourself and your body.

Promotes relaxation

Physical activity and exercise can help to relax the mind and body, making it a great way to unwind after a long day.

By taking care of your physical health, you can also benefit your mental health and overall well-being. So, make time for physical activity and exercise, and enjoy the many physical and mental benefits it has to offer.

Stretching as a Form of Stress Relief and Relaxation: The Benefits of Taking a Few Minutes to Stretch

Stretching is a simple, yet effective way to reduce stress and relax the mind and body

Behaviors in which stretching can help to relieve stress and promote relaxation

Releases tension

Stretching helps to release tension in the muscles, which can help to alleviate stress and promote relaxation.

Focuses the mind

Stretching requires you to focus on your breath and the sensation of stretching, which can help to calm the mind and promote relaxation.

Increases mindfulness

By focusing on the present moment, stretching can help to increase mindfulness and improve overall well-being.

Promotes relaxation

Stretching can help to relax the mind and body, making it a great way to unwind after a long day.

By taking a few minutes to stretch each day, you can enjoy the many physical and mental benefits it has to offer. Remember to listen to your body and only do stretches that feel comfortable for you. With regular practice, stretching can be an effective way to reduce stress and promote relaxation.

Techniques for Incorporating Mindful Breathing and Meditation into Your Stretching Routine

Incorporating mindful breathing and meditation into your stretching routine can help to increase relaxation and improve overall well-being. Here are a few techniques you can try:

Focus on your breath

As you stretch, focus on your breath and the sensation of stretching. Try to take slow, deep breaths and let your breath guide your movements.

Use visualization

As you stretch, try to visualize yourself in a peaceful, calming place. This can help to relax the mind and promote a sense of calm.

Set an intention

Before you begin stretching, try setting an intention for your practice. It can be as simple as "I am releasing tension and relaxing my mind and body." This can help to focus the mind and improve the effectiveness of your stretches.

Practice gratitude

As you stretch, try to focus on the things you are grateful for. This can help to shift your focus away from stress and promote a sense of well-being.

By incorporating mindful breathing and meditation into your stretching routine, you can increase relaxation and improve overall well-being. Remember to take it easy and only do stretches that feel comfortable for you. With regular practice, these techniques can help to improve relaxation and promote a sense of calm and well-being.